THE ANKYLOSING SPONDYLITIS DIET BIBLE

Integrating Science And Nutrition To Alleviate Symptoms And Implement Dietary Strategies To Promote Joint Health And Reduce Pain

CRUE GAGE

Table of Contents

Introductory

Ankylosing spondylitis (AS) is a form of inflammatory arthritis that predominantly impacts the sacroiliac joints in the pelvis and the spine. Over time, it may cause the vertebrae in the spine to fuse together, resulting in reduced flexibility and a hunched posture, as well as discomfort and stiffness in the back and hips.

Chronic pain is a common symptom, particularly in the lower back and pelvis, and it may be alleviated by physical activity. Although the precise cause remains unclear, genetic factors, particularly the HLA-B27 gene, are suspected to be involved.

Symptom management is the primary objective of treatment, which may involve lifestyle modifications, physical therapy, and medications.

Symptoms And Diagnosis

Symptoms of Ankylosing Spondylitis:

- **Chronic Back Pain**: Typically starts in the lower back and can improve with activity but worsens with rest.

- **Stiffness**: Especially noticeable in the morning or after periods of inactivity.

- **Pain in Other Joints**: May affect hips, shoulders, and knees.

- **Fatigue**: Due to chronic inflammation.

- **Reduced Flexibility**: Over time, spinal mobility may decrease.

- **Posture Changes**: Can lead to a stooped or hunched posture as the disease progresses.
- **Eye Inflammation**: Some patients experience uveitis, leading to eye pain and redness.

Diagnosis:

- **Medical History and Symptoms**: A doctor will assess the patient's history and symptom patterns.
- **Physical Examination**: Evaluating the range of motion, posture, and tenderness in the spine and joints.

Imaging Tests:

- **X-rays**: To detect changes in the spine and pelvis.

- **MRI**: Can show early signs of inflammation in the sacroiliac joints.

- **Blood Tests**: Checking for the HLA-B27 antigen and markers of inflammation (such as C-reactive protein or ESR).

Early diagnosis and treatment are important to manage symptoms and slow disease progression.

CHAPTER ONE
Causes & Risk Factors

Causes of Ankylosing Spondylitis:

The exact cause of ankylosing spondylitis (AS) is not fully understood, but it is believed to be related to a combination of genetic, environmental, and immune system factors. The condition is associated with chronic inflammation that affects the spine and joints.

Risk Factors:

Genetics:

• **HLA-B27 Antigen**: A significant risk factor; having this antigen increases the likelihood of developing AS, though not everyone with the antigen will develop the disease.

Family History:

• A family history of ankylosing spondylitis or related autoimmune conditions increases risk.

Age:

• AS typically begins in late adolescence or early adulthood, though it can develop at any age.

Gender:

• More common in males than females, often with more severe symptoms in men.

Other Conditions:

• Individuals with other autoimmune conditions (like psoriasis or inflammatory bowel disease) may have a higher risk.

Environmental Factors:

• Some studies suggest that infections or certain environmental triggers might play a role, although more research is needed.

While having one or more risk factors can increase the likelihood of developing AS, not everyone with these factors will experience the disease.

Traditional Treatments And Lifestyle Changes

Traditional Treatments for Ankylosing Spondylitis:

Medications:

• **Nonsteroidal Anti-Inflammatory Drugs (NSAIDs)**: Help reduce pain and inflammation (e.g., ibuprofen, naproxen).

- **Disease-Modifying Antirheumatic Drugs (DMARDs)**: May be used if NSAIDs are ineffective (e.g., sulfasalazine).

- **Biologic Medications**: Target specific components of the immune system (e.g., TNF inhibitors like etanercept, infliximab, and IL-17 inhibitors).

- **Corticosteroids**: Used in flare-ups to reduce inflammation.

<u>**Physical Therapy**</u>:

• Tailored exercises to improve flexibility and posture, along with stretching to maintain spinal mobility.

Pain Management:

• Techniques such as heat therapy, cold packs, and acupuncture may be helpful.

Surgery:

- In severe cases, surgical intervention may be needed to correct significant spinal deformities or joint damage.

<u>Lifestyle Changes:</u>

Regular Exercise:

- Engaging in low-impact activities (like swimming, walking, or cycling) helps maintain flexibility and strength.

Posture Awareness:

- Practicing good posture can help alleviate discomfort and prevent worsening of spinal curvature.

Healthy Diet:

- A balanced diet rich in anti-inflammatory foods (such as fruits, vegetables, and omega-3 fatty acids) may help reduce inflammation.

Weight Management:

• Maintaining a healthy weight can reduce stress on the joints.

Smoking Cessation:

• Quitting smoking can improve overall health and reduce the risk of complications.

Stress Management:

• Techniques like mindfulness, yoga, and meditation may help manage pain and improve overall well-being.

Incorporating these treatments and lifestyle changes can significantly improve quality of life for individuals with ankylosing spondylitis. Always consult with a healthcare provider for a personalized treatment plan.

Importance Of Diet In Managing Ankylosing Spondylitis (AS)

Inflammation Reduction:

• A healthy diet can help lower systemic inflammation, potentially alleviating symptoms. Foods rich in antioxidants, such as fruits and vegetables, are particularly beneficial.

Weight Management:

• Maintaining a healthy weight reduces stress on the joints and spine, which can help decrease pain and improve mobility.

Nutrient Intake:

• A balanced diet ensures adequate intake of essential nutrients that support overall health, including vitamins and minerals that may have anti-inflammatory properties (e.g., omega-3 fatty acids, vitamin D, and calcium).

Gut Health:

• Some studies suggest a link between gut health and inflammatory diseases. A diet rich in fiber and probiotics can promote a healthy gut microbiome, potentially impacting inflammation.

Consulting with a healthcare provider or nutritionist can help develop a personalized dietary plan that aligns with managing AS effectively.

Key Nutritional Needs For AS Patients

Key Nutritional Needs for Ankylosing Spondylitis (AS) Patients

Omega-3 Fatty Acids:

• Found in fatty fish (like salmon and mackerel), flaxseeds, and walnuts, omega-3s have anti-inflammatory properties that can help reduce joint inflammation.

Vitamin D:

• Essential for bone health and immune function. Sources include sunlight, fortified foods, and fatty fish. Supplements may be necessary for those with low levels.

Calcium:

• Important for bone health, especially as AS can lead to spinal issues. Dairy products, leafy greens, and fortified foods are good sources.

Magnesium:

• Plays a role in muscle and nerve function, and can be found in nuts, seeds, whole grains, and leafy greens.

Antioxidants:

• Vitamins A, C, and E, as well as selenium, help combat oxidative stress. These can be obtained from a variety of fruits, vegetables, nuts, and seeds.

Fiber:

• Aids in digestion and gut health. Whole grains, fruits, vegetables, and legumes are rich sources of fiber.

Probiotics:

• Beneficial for gut health. Found in yogurt, kefir, sauerkraut, and other fermented foods.

Hydration:

• Staying well-hydrated is important for overall health and can help manage inflammation.

A well-rounded diet that incorporates these nutrients can support overall health and help manage symptoms of ankylosing spondylitis. Always consider consulting with a healthcare provider or nutritionist for tailored dietary advice.

CHAPTER TWO
How Diet Affects Inflammation

Diet can significantly affect inflammation in the body, impacting conditions like ankylosing spondylitis (AS). Here's how:

• Certain foods contain compounds that help reduce inflammation. For example, omega-3 fatty acids found in fatty fish, flaxseeds, and walnuts can lower inflammatory markers in the body.

• Foods rich in antioxidants (like fruits and vegetables) help combat oxidative stress, which is linked to chronic inflammation. Vitamins A, C, and E, as well as phytochemicals, play a protective role.

• Healthy fats (such as those from olive oil, avocados, and nuts) can reduce inflammation, while trans fats and excessive saturated fats can promote it.

• Diets high in processed foods, refined sugars, and carbohydrates can lead to increased inflammation. These foods can trigger the release of inflammatory cytokines.

• A diet rich in fiber and probiotics supports gut health, which is increasingly recognized for its role in regulating inflammation. A healthy gut microbiome can modulate immune responses.

• Some individuals may have specific food sensitivities (e.g., gluten, dairy) that can trigger inflammatory responses. Identifying and eliminating these foods can help reduce inflammation.

• A whole-foods-based diet, emphasizing fresh, minimally processed foods, tends to be associated with lower inflammation compared to a diet high in processed foods.

By adopting an anti-inflammatory diet, individuals can potentially manage symptoms and improve overall health, especially in conditions characterized by chronic inflammation like AS.

Top Anti-Inflammatory Foods

Here are some top anti-inflammatory foods that can help reduce inflammation and support overall health:

• **Fatty Fish**: Salmon, mackerel, sardines, and trout are rich in omega-3 fatty acids, which have strong anti-inflammatory properties.

• **Fruits**: Berries (such as blueberries, strawberries, and raspberries), cherries, and oranges are high in antioxidants and vitamins that combat inflammation.

• **Leafy Greens**: Spinach, kale, and Swiss chard are packed with vitamins, minerals, and antioxidants that can help lower inflammation.

• **Nuts and Seeds**: Almonds, walnuts, flaxseeds, and chia seeds are good sources of healthy fats and omega-3s.

• **Olive Oil**: Extra virgin olive oil contains oleocanthal, a compound with anti-inflammatory effects similar to ibuprofen.

• **Turmeric**: Curcumin, the active compound in turmeric, has powerful anti-inflammatory and antioxidant properties.

- **Ginger**: Known for its anti-inflammatory effects, ginger can be consumed fresh, in teas, or as a spice in cooking.

- **Garlic**: Contains compounds that can enhance the immune system and reduce inflammation.

- **Whole Grains**: Foods like oats, quinoa, and brown rice are high in fiber, which can help reduce inflammation.

- **Legumes**: Beans, lentils, and chickpeas are rich in fiber and protein, contributing to overall health and reduced inflammation.

Incorporating these foods into your diet can help manage inflammation and improve overall well-being.

Foods To Avoid

Here are some foods to avoid to help reduce inflammation:

• **Processed Foods**: Foods high in refined sugars and unhealthy fats, such as chips, cookies, and packaged snacks, can promote inflammation.

• **Sugary Beverages**: Soft drinks, energy drinks, and high-sugar fruit juices can increase inflammatory markers in the body.

• **Refined Carbohydrates**: White bread, pastries, and other foods made with white flour can spike blood sugar and contribute to inflammation.

• **Trans Fats**: Found in some fried foods, baked goods, and margarine, trans fats are linked to increased inflammation and heart disease.

• **Excessive Alcohol**: High alcohol consumption can trigger inflammatory responses and negatively impact gut health.

• **Red and Processed Meats**: These can contain high levels of saturated fats and compounds that promote inflammation, especially processed meats like sausages and hot dogs.

• **High-Sodium Foods**: Excessive salt can lead to increased blood pressure and inflammation, commonly found in processed and canned foods.

• **Dairy (for some individuals)**: Some people may have sensitivities to dairy products, which can lead to increased inflammation.

• **Certain Oils**: Vegetable oils high in omega-6 fatty acids (like corn and soybean oil) can promote inflammation when consumed in excess relative to omega-3s.

Avoiding these foods can help manage inflammation and improve overall health, especially for individuals with conditions like ankylosing spondylitis.

<h2 style="text-align:center">Breakfast Recipes</h2>

Here are some healthy breakfast recipes that incorporate anti-inflammatory ingredients:

1. Overnight Oats:

Ingredients:

- 1/2 cup rolled oats
- 1 cup almond milk (or your choice)
- 1 tablespoon chia seeds
- 1 tablespoon honey or maple syrup
- Fresh berries (blueberries, strawberries)
- A sprinkle of cinnamon

Instructions:

- In a jar or bowl, combine oats, almond milk, chia seeds, and honey.
- Mix well and refrigerate overnight.
- In the morning, top with fresh berries and a sprinkle of cinnamon.

2. Avocado Toast with Poached Egg:

Ingredients:

- 1 slice whole-grain bread
- 1/2 ripe avocado
- 1 egg
- Salt and pepper to taste
- Red pepper flakes (optional)
- Fresh lemon juice

Instructions:

- Toast the bread until golden.
- Mash the avocado with a squeeze of lemon juice, salt, and pepper.
- Poach the egg in simmering water for about 3-4 minutes.
- Spread the avocado on the toast, top with the poached egg, and sprinkle with red pepper flakes if desired.

3. Smoothie Bowl:

Ingredients:

- 1 banana
- 1/2 cup spinach
- 1/2 cup frozen berries (blueberries, strawberries)
- 1 tablespoon flaxseeds
- 1 cup almond milk (or yogurt)

- Toppings: sliced fruit, nuts, seeds, granola

Instructions:

- Blend the banana, spinach, frozen berries, flaxseeds, and almond milk until smooth.
- Pour into a bowl and top with your choice of sliced fruit, nuts, seeds, and granola.

4. Chia Seed Pudding:

Ingredients:

- 1/4 cup chia seeds
- 1 cup almond milk (or any milk)
- 1 tablespoon maple syrup or honey
- 1/2 teaspoon vanilla extract
- Fresh fruit for topping (mango, berries, etc.)

Instructions:

- In a bowl, mix chia seeds, almond milk, sweetener, and vanilla extract.
- Stir well and refrigerate for at least 2 hours or overnight.
- Serve topped with fresh fruit.

5. Veggie Omelette:

Ingredients:

- 2 eggs (or egg whites)
- Spinach, bell peppers, onions, and tomatoes (or any veggies you like)
- Salt and pepper to taste
- Olive oil or cooking spray

Instructions:

- Whisk the eggs in a bowl and season with salt and pepper.

- Heat a non-stick skillet over medium heat with a little olive oil.

- Sauté the veggies until tender, then pour the eggs over them.

- Cook until the edges are set, then fold and serve.

These recipes are nutritious, easy to prepare, and packed with anti-inflammatory ingredients!

Lunch Recipes

Here are some healthy lunch recipes that incorporate anti-inflammatory ingredients:

1. Quinoa Salad Bowl:

Ingredients:

- 1 cup cooked quinoa

- 1/2 cup cherry tomatoes, halved

- 1/2 cucumber, diced

- 1/4 red onion, diced
- 1/4 cup chickpeas (canned, rinsed)
- Fresh parsley or cilantro, chopped
- Lemon juice, olive oil, salt, and pepper to taste

Instructions:

- In a large bowl, combine cooked quinoa, cherry tomatoes, cucumber, red onion, chickpeas, and herbs.
- Drizzle with lemon juice and olive oil, then season with salt and pepper. Toss to combine.

2. Mediterranean Chickpea Wrap:

Ingredients:

- Whole-grain wrap or pita
- 1/2 cup canned chickpeas, rinsed

- 1/4 avocado, sliced

- Spinach or mixed greens

- Sliced cucumber and bell pepper

- Hummus

- Olive oil, lemon juice, and salt for dressing

Instructions:

- Spread hummus on the wrap.

- Layer with spinach, chickpeas, avocado, cucumber, and bell pepper.

- Drizzle with olive oil and lemon juice, season with salt, then roll up the wrap and enjoy.

3. Lentil Soup:

Ingredients:

- 1 cup lentils, rinsed

- 1 onion, diced

- 2 carrots, diced

- 2 celery stalks, diced

- 3 cloves garlic, minced

- 4 cups vegetable broth

- 1 teaspoon cumin

- 1 teaspoon turmeric

- Salt and pepper to taste

- Fresh parsley for garnish

Instructions:

- In a large pot, sauté onion, carrots, celery, and garlic until softened.

- Add lentils, vegetable broth, cumin, turmeric, salt, and pepper.

- Bring to a boil, then reduce heat and simmer for about 30-40 minutes, until lentils are tender.

- Serve hot, garnished with fresh parsley.

4. Sweet Potato and Black Bean Bowl:

Ingredients:

- 1 medium sweet potato, diced
- 1 can black beans, rinsed
- 1 avocado, diced
- 1 cup cooked brown rice or quinoa
- Spinach or kale
- Lime juice, cumin, and chili powder for seasoning

Instructions:

- Roast diced sweet potato in the oven at 400°F (200°C) for 20-25 minutes until tender.
- In a bowl, layer cooked brown rice or quinoa, roasted sweet potato, black beans, and greens.
- Top with avocado and season with lime juice, cumin, and chili powder.

5. Spinach and Feta Stuffed Chicken Breast:

Ingredients:

- 2 boneless chicken breasts
- 1 cup fresh spinach, sautéed
- 1/4 cup feta cheese, crumbled
- 1 tablespoon olive oil
- Salt, pepper, and garlic powder to taste

Instructions:

- Preheat the oven to 375°F (190°C).
- Cut a pocket in each chicken breast and stuff with sautéed spinach and feta.
- Season with salt, pepper, and garlic powder, then drizzle with olive oil.

- Bake for 25-30 minutes, until chicken is cooked through.

These recipes are not only delicious but also packed with nutrients that can help combat inflammation!

Dinner Dishes Recipes

Here are some healthy dinner recipes featuring anti-inflammatory ingredients:

1. Baked Salmon with Asparagus:

Ingredients:

- 2 salmon fillets
- 1 bunch asparagus, trimmed
- 2 tablespoons olive oil
- 2 cloves garlic, minced
- Lemon slices
- Salt and pepper to taste

Instructions:

- Preheat the oven to 400°F (200°C).
- Place salmon fillets and asparagus on a baking sheet. Drizzle with olive oil, garlic, salt, and pepper.
- Top salmon with lemon slices.
- Bake for about 15-20 minutes, until salmon is cooked through and asparagus is tender.

2. Chickpea and Spinach Curry:

Ingredients:

- 1 can chickpeas, rinsed
- 2 cups fresh spinach
- 1 onion, diced
- 2 cloves garlic, minced
- 1 tablespoon ginger, minced
- 1 can coconut milk
- 1 tablespoon curry powder
- 1 tablespoon olive oil

- Salt to taste

Instructions:

- Heat olive oil in a large pan. Sauté onion, garlic, and ginger until softened.
- Add curry powder and cook for 1 minute.
- Stir in chickpeas and coconut milk. Simmer for about 10 minutes.
- Add spinach and cook until wilted. Season with salt and serve with brown rice or quinoa.

3. Stuffed Bell Peppers:

Ingredients:

- 4 bell peppers, halved and seeded
- 1 cup cooked quinoa
- 1 can black beans, rinsed
- 1 cup corn (fresh or frozen)

- 1 teaspoon cumin

- 1 teaspoon chili powder

- Salt and pepper to taste

- Shredded cheese (optional)

Instructions:

- Preheat the oven to 375°F (190°C).

- In a bowl, mix cooked quinoa, black beans, corn, cumin, chili powder, salt, and pepper.

- Stuff the mixture into halved bell peppers.

- Place in a baking dish and bake for 25-30 minutes. Top with cheese during the last 5 minutes if desired.

4. Zucchini Noodles with Pesto and Cherry Tomatoes:

Ingredients:

- 2 medium zucchinis, spiralized

- 1 cup cherry tomatoes, halved

- 1/4 cup pesto (store-bought or homemade)

- 2 tablespoons olive oil

- Salt and pepper to taste

Instructions:

- In a large skillet, heat olive oil over medium heat.

- Add cherry tomatoes and sauté for 3-4 minutes until softened.

- Add zucchini noodles and cook for another 2-3 minutes.

- Stir in pesto and season with salt and pepper. Serve immediately.

5. Turkey and Vegetable Stir-Fry:

Ingredients:

- 1 pound ground turkey

- 2 cups mixed vegetables (broccoli, bell peppers, snap peas)
- 2 cloves garlic, minced
- 1 tablespoon ginger, minced
- 2 tablespoons soy sauce (or tamari for gluten-free)
- 1 tablespoon sesame oil

Instructions:

- In a large skillet or wok, heat sesame oil over medium heat.
- Add ground turkey and cook until browned.
- Add garlic, ginger, and mixed vegetables. Stir-fry for about 5-7 minutes.
- Stir in soy sauce and cook for an additional 2 minutes. Serve hot.

These dinner recipes are nutritious, delicious, and perfect for an anti-inflammatory diet! Enjoy!

Snack & Desserts Recipes

Here are some healthy snack and dessert recipes featuring anti-inflammatory ingredients:

Snacks:

1. Hummus and Veggies:

Ingredients:

- 1 can chickpeas, rinsed
- 2 tablespoons tahini
- 2 tablespoons olive oil
- 1 clove garlic, minced
- Juice of 1 lemon
- Salt and pepper to taste

- Fresh veggies (carrots, cucumbers, bell peppers) for dipping

Instructions:

- In a food processor, combine chickpeas, tahini, olive oil, garlic, lemon juice, salt, and pepper.
- Blend until smooth, adding water if needed for desired consistency.
- Serve with fresh veggies for dipping.

2. Nut and Seed Energy Balls:

Ingredients:

- 1 cup mixed nuts (almonds, walnuts, cashews)
- 1/2 cup rolled oats
- 1/4 cup nut butter (almond or peanut)
- 1/4 cup honey or maple syrup

- 1/4 cup flaxseeds or chia seeds
- 1/4 cup dark chocolate chips (optional)

Instructions:

- In a bowl, mix all ingredients until well combined.
- Roll the mixture into small balls and place on a baking sheet.
- Refrigerate for at least 30 minutes to firm up. Store in the fridge.

Desserts:

3. Chia Seed Pudding with Berries:

Ingredients:

- 1/4 cup chia seeds
- 1 cup almond milk (or other milk)
- 1 tablespoon maple syrup or honey

- 1/2 teaspoon vanilla extract

- Fresh berries for topping

Instructions:

- In a bowl, mix chia seeds, almond milk, maple syrup, and vanilla.

- Stir well and refrigerate for at least 2 hours or overnight.

- Serve topped with fresh berries.

4. Banana Oat Cookies:

Ingredients:

- 2 ripe bananas, mashed

- 1 cup rolled oats

- 1/2 teaspoon cinnamon

- 1/4 cup dark chocolate chips or nuts (optional)

Instructions:

- Preheat the oven to 350°F (175°C).

- In a bowl, mix mashed bananas, oats, and cinnamon until combined. Stir in chocolate chips or nuts if desired.
- Drop spoonfuls of the mixture onto a baking sheet lined with parchment paper.
- Bake for 12-15 minutes until lightly golden. Let cool before serving.

5. Baked Apples with Cinnamon:

Ingredients:

- 4 apples, cored
- 1/4 cup rolled oats
- 1 tablespoon honey or maple syrup
- 1 teaspoon cinnamon
- 1/4 cup walnuts or pecans, chopped (optional)

Instructions:

- Preheat the oven to 350°F (175°C).

- In a bowl, mix oats, honey, cinnamon, and nuts.

- Stuff the mixture into the cored apples and place in a baking dish.

- Bake for 25-30 minutes until apples are tender. Serve warm.

These snacks and desserts are delicious and packed with nutrients, making them great choices for an anti-inflammatory diet! Enjoy!

CHAPTER THREE

Herbal Supplements And Their Benefits

Here are some common herbal supplements and their potential benefits:

1. Turmeric (Curcumin):

- **Benefits**: Known for its anti-inflammatory properties, turmeric may help reduce inflammation, alleviate joint pain, and support digestive health. Curcumin, the active compound, is often highlighted for its potential effects on chronic inflammation and oxidative stress.

2. Ginger:

- **Benefits**: Ginger may help reduce muscle pain and soreness, particularly related to exercise. It has anti-inflammatory and antioxidant effects, which can support digestive health and alleviate nausea.

3. Boswellia (Frankincense):

- **Benefits**: Boswellia extract is known for its anti-inflammatory properties and may be effective in managing conditions like arthritis. It may help reduce joint pain and improve mobility.

4. Green Tea Extract:

- **Benefits**: Rich in antioxidants, particularly catechins, green tea extract may help reduce inflammation, support heart health, and improve metabolic function. It may also have benefits for brain health.

5. Willow Bark:

• **Benefits**: Traditionally used for pain relief, willow bark contains salicin, which is similar to aspirin. It may help reduce pain and inflammation, particularly in conditions like osteoarthritis and lower back pain.

6. Milk Thistle (Silymarin):

Benefits: Milk thistle is often used to support liver health. Silymarin, its active component, has antioxidant and anti-inflammatory properties that may help protect liver cells.

7. Devil's Claw:

• **Benefits**: Commonly used for pain relief, especially in osteoarthritis and back pain, devil's claw may help reduce inflammation and improve joint function.

8. Ashwagandha:

- **Benefits**: An adaptogen that may help reduce stress and anxiety, ashwagandha can also support immune function and has anti-inflammatory effects. It may help improve energy levels and overall well-being.

9. Echinacea:

- **Benefits**: Often used to boost the immune system, echinacea may help reduce the duration and severity of colds and respiratory infections.

10. Rhodiola Rosea:

- **Benefits**: This adaptogen may help reduce fatigue and improve mental performance, particularly in stressful situations. It may also have anti-inflammatory properties.

<u>**Important Considerations:**</u>

• **Consult a Healthcare Provider**: Always talk to a healthcare professional before starting any new supplement, especially if you have underlying health conditions or are taking medications.

• **Quality Matters**: Choose high-quality supplements from reputable brands to ensure potency and safety.

How To Incorporate Supplements Safely

Incorporating herbal supplements safely involves several important steps:

• Discuss any supplements you're considering with your healthcare provider, especially if you have existing health conditions or are on medication. A registered dietitian or nutritionist can help tailor supplement choices to your specific needs.

• Familiarize yourself with the potential benefits, side effects, and interactions of the supplements you're considering. Look for supplements that have been third-party tested for quality and potency (look for certifications like USP or NSF).

• This helps you monitor for any adverse reactions or side effects. Adhere to the recommended dosage on the label or as advised by your healthcare provider.

• Track how you feel after starting a new supplement. Note any changes in health, mood, or energy levels. Be aware of potential interactions with medications or other supplements you may be taking.

• Aim to get nutrients from a balanced diet before relying on supplements. Supplements are meant to complement, not replace, a healthy diet.

• Periodically review whether you still need the supplement based on changes in your health, diet, or lifestyle. If you experience any health changes or are considering new supplements, consult your healthcare provider.

• Store supplements in a cool, dark place to maintain potency. Always check the expiration date and discard any expired products.

By following these guidelines, you can incorporate herbal supplements safely and effectively into your health routine.

Creating A 7 Days Balanced Meal Plan

Here's a 7-day balanced meal plan featuring a variety of nutrients and anti-inflammatory foods. Adjust portion sizes based on your individual needs.

Day 1:

- **Breakfast**: Overnight oats with chia seeds, almond milk, and fresh berries.

- **Lunch**: Quinoa salad with cherry tomatoes, cucumber, chickpeas, and a lemon-olive oil dressing.
- **Snack**: Hummus with carrot and cucumber sticks.
- **Dinner**: Baked salmon with asparagus and a side of brown rice.

Day 2:

- **Breakfast**: Smoothie with spinach, banana, almond milk, and a tablespoon of flaxseeds.
- **Lunch**: Whole-grain wrap with turkey, avocado, spinach, and hummus.
- **Snack**: A handful of mixed nuts.
- **Dinner**: Chickpea and spinach curry served with quinoa.

Day 3:

- **Breakfast**: Scrambled eggs with sautéed kale and tomatoes.
- **Lunch**: Lentil soup with whole-grain bread.
- **Snack**: Apple slices with almond butter.
- **Dinner**: Stuffed bell peppers with quinoa, black beans, and spices.

Day 4:

- **Breakfast**: Greek yogurt with honey, walnuts, and sliced banana.
- **Lunch**: Spinach and feta salad with grilled chicken and vinaigrette.
- **Snack**: Celery sticks with peanut butter.
- **Dinner**: Zucchini noodles with pesto and cherry tomatoes.

Day 5:

- **Breakfast**: Chia seed pudding topped with fresh fruit.
- **Lunch**: Mediterranean bowl with farro, olives, roasted vegetables, and feta cheese.
- **Snack**: Sliced bell peppers with guacamole.
- **Dinner**: Grilled shrimp with quinoa and steamed broccoli.

Day 6:

- **Breakfast**: Whole-grain toast with avocado and poached egg.
- **Lunch**: Turkey and vegetable stir-fry with brown rice.
- **Snack**: A small handful of dried fruit and seeds.
- **Dinner**: Baked chicken thighs with sweet potatoes and green beans.

Day 7:

- **Breakfast**: Oatmeal with cinnamon, apple slices, and walnuts.

- **Lunch**: Black bean salad with corn, diced peppers, and lime dressing.

- **Snack**: Greek yogurt with a sprinkle of cinnamon.

- **Dinner**: Vegetable stir-fry with tofu, served over brown rice.

Tips:

- **Hydration**: Drink plenty of water throughout the day.

- **Adjust Portions**: Modify portion sizes and snacks according to your energy needs.

- **Prep Ahead**: Meal prep ingredients in advance to save time during the week.

Feel free to swap meals and snacks as desired to keep things interesting!

CHAPTER FOUR
Grocery Shopping Tips

Here are some practical grocery shopping tips to help you make healthier choices:

1. Plan Your Meals:

• **Create a Meal Plan**: Before shopping, plan your meals for the week. This helps you know what ingredients you need and reduces impulse purchases.

• **Make a Shopping List**: Write down the items you need based on your meal plan to stay focused and avoid buying unnecessary items.

2. Shop the Perimeter:

• **Focus on Fresh Foods**: The perimeter of the store typically has fresh produce, dairy, meats, and whole grains. These are often healthier choices compared to processed foods found in the center aisles.

3. Choose Whole Foods:

• **Opt for Whole Grains**: Look for brown rice, quinoa, whole-grain bread, and oats instead of refined grains.

• **Select Fresh or Frozen Produce**: Fresh fruits and vegetables are great, but frozen options without added sugar or sauces can be just as nutritious and convenient.

4. Read Labels:

• **Check Ingredients**: Look for items with minimal ingredients and avoid those with added sugars, preservatives, and unhealthy fats.

• **Watch for Serving Sizes**: Pay attention to serving sizes on nutrition labels to better understand portion control.

5. Buy in Bulk:

• **Stock Up on Staples**: Consider buying grains, legumes, nuts, and seeds in bulk to save money and reduce packaging waste.

• **Choose Freezer-Friendly Items**: Purchase frozen fruits and vegetables in bulk for easy access and longer shelf life.

6. Be Mindful of Sales:

• **Look for Discounts**: Keep an eye out for sales, but be cautious of purchasing items just because they are on sale. Stick to your list.

• **Use Coupons Wisely**: If you use coupons, make sure they are for items you actually need and use.

7. Stay Hydrated and Snack Smart:

• **Don't Shop Hungry**: Eating a healthy snack before grocery shopping can help you avoid impulse buys of unhealthy snacks.

• **Plan for Healthy Snacks**: Include items like fruits, nuts, and yogurt on your list for nutritious snacking.

8. Try New Things:

• **Explore New Ingredients**: Don't hesitate to try new fruits, vegetables, or whole grains to keep your meals interesting and varied.

By following these tips, you can make healthier choices, save money, and streamline your grocery shopping experience!

Batch Cooking And Freezing

Batch cooking and freezing are excellent strategies for saving time and ensuring you have healthy meals ready when needed. Here are some tips on how to effectively batch cook and freeze meals:

Tips for Batch Cooking:

• Choose recipes that store well and can be easily reheated. Plan a variety of meals to keep your menu interesting.

• Dedicate a few hours on a weekend or a day off to cook in bulk. Gather all ingredients and cooking tools before starting.

• Cook larger quantities of grains, legumes, and proteins that can be used in different meals throughout the week.

• Chop vegetables, marinate proteins, or pre-cook grains ahead of time to save prep time during cooking.

• Use multiple pots and pans to cook different items simultaneously. Consider using a slow cooker or pressure cooker for easy meal preparation.

<u>Freezing Tips:</u>

• Allow cooked meals to cool before freezing to prevent ice crystals and maintain texture.

• Store meals in freezer-safe, airtight containers or heavy-duty freezer bags to prevent freezer burn. Label containers with the name of the dish and the date prepared.

• Freeze meals in single-serving or family-sized portions based on your needs. Consider freezing ingredients separately (e.g., cooked grains and vegetables) for easy mixing later.

• Most cooked meals can be frozen for up to 3 months without losing quality. However, they are best consumed sooner for optimal taste.

• Thaw meals in the refrigerator overnight for safe reheating. For quick reheating, you can use the microwave or stovetop. Ensure food is heated to at least 165°F (74°C) before consuming.

Meal Ideas for Batch Cooking and Freezing:

- **Soups and Stews**: These freeze well and can be portioned for easy meals.

- **Chili**: A hearty option that can be made in bulk and frozen.

- **Casseroles**: Layered dishes like lasagna or baked pasta freeze nicely.

- **Cooked Grains**: Brown rice, quinoa, or barley can be cooked in bulk and frozen for quick meal prep.

- **Stir-fried Vegetables**: Pre-cook a variety of vegetables that can be used in stir-fries or as side dishes.

By batch cooking and freezing meals, you can save time, reduce stress during busy weeks, and maintain a healthy diet!

Tips For Dining Out

Dining out can be enjoyable while still adhering to healthy eating habits. Here are some tips to make nutritious choices when eating at restaurants:

1. Check the Menu Ahead of Time:

• **Review Options**: Look at the restaurant's menu online to identify healthy options before you arrive.

• **Make Reservations**: This can help reduce wait times and ensure a more relaxed dining experience.

2. Choose Wisely:

• **Select Whole Foods**: Opt for dishes that include whole grains, lean proteins, and plenty of vegetables.

- **Avoid Fried Foods**: Choose grilled, baked, or steamed options over fried ones to reduce unhealthy fats.

3. Control Portions:

- **Share Dishes**: Consider sharing an appetizer or dessert with someone to enjoy variety without overindulging.

- **Request Smaller Portions**: Many restaurants offer lunch-sized portions or you can ask for half portions.

4. Customize Your Order:

- **Modify Ingredients**: Don't hesitate to ask for dressings or sauces on the side, substitute fries with a side salad, or request whole-grain options if available.

- **Limit High-Calorie Add-ons**: Be mindful of cheese, cream sauces, and excessive toppings that can add unnecessary calories.

5. Start with a Salad or Soup:

• **Order a Salad**: Starting with a salad (dressing on the side) can help fill you up with fiber and nutrients, making it easier to manage portion sizes for the main course.

• **Opt for Broth-Based Soups**: These can be lighter and lower in calories compared to creamy soups.

6. Stay Hydrated:

• **Drink Water**: Opt for water or unsweetened beverages instead of sugary sodas or alcohol to reduce calorie intake.

• **Limit Alcohol**: If you choose to drink, do so in moderation, as alcoholic beverages can add significant calories.

7. Listen to Your Body:

• **Eat Mindfully**: Pay attention to your hunger cues and eat slowly to allow your body time to signal fullness.

• **Take Leftovers**: If you find yourself with too much food, don't hesitate to take leftovers home for another meal.

8. Be Cautious with Desserts:

• **Share Desserts**: If you want dessert, consider sharing it to satisfy your sweet tooth without overdoing it.

• **Choose Fruit-Based Options**: If available, opt for fruit-based desserts or sorbets for a lighter finish.

By applying these tips, you can enjoy dining out while making healthier choices that align with your dietary goals!

CHAPTER FIVE
Gluten-Free Diet Anti-Inflammatory Recipes

Here are some delicious gluten-free recipes that are also anti-inflammatory:

1. Quinoa and Black Bean Salad:

Ingredients:

- 1 cup cooked quinoa
- 1 can black beans, rinsed
- 1 bell pepper, diced
- 1 cup corn (fresh or frozen)
- 1/4 cup cilantro, chopped
- Juice of 1 lime
- 2 tablespoons olive oil
- Salt and pepper to taste

Instructions:

- In a large bowl, combine quinoa, black beans, bell pepper, corn, and cilantro.
- Drizzle with lime juice and olive oil, then season with salt and pepper. Toss to combine and serve chilled.

2. Zucchini Noodles with Pesto:

Ingredients:

- 2 medium zucchinis, spiralized
- 1/2 cup basil pesto (store-bought or homemade)
- 1 cup cherry tomatoes, halved
- 2 tablespoons olive oil
- Salt and pepper to taste

Instructions:

- Heat olive oil in a skillet over medium heat. Add zucchini noodles and sauté for 2-3 minutes until slightly softened.
- Stir in cherry tomatoes and pesto, cooking for another minute.
- Season with salt and pepper, then serve immediately.

<u>3. Turmeric Roasted Cauliflower:</u>

Ingredients:

- 1 head cauliflower, cut into florets
- 2 tablespoons olive oil
- 1 teaspoon turmeric powder
- 1 teaspoon cumin
- Salt and pepper to taste

Instructions:

- Preheat the oven to 425°F (220°C).

- In a bowl, toss cauliflower florets with olive oil, turmeric, cumin, salt, and pepper until well coated.

- Spread on a baking sheet and roast for 25-30 minutes, until golden brown and tender.

4. Chickpea and Spinach Stew:

Ingredients:

- 1 can chickpeas, rinsed

- 2 cups fresh spinach

- 1 onion, diced

- 2 cloves garlic, minced

- 1 can diced tomatoes

- 1 teaspoon cumin

- 1 teaspoon paprika

- Olive oil, salt, and pepper to taste

Instructions:

- Heat olive oil in a pot over medium heat. Sauté onion and garlic until softened.

- Add chickpeas, diced tomatoes, cumin, and paprika. Simmer for 10 minutes.

- Stir in fresh spinach until wilted, then season with salt and pepper. Serve warm.

5. Berry Chia Seed Pudding:

Ingredients:

- 1/4 cup chia seeds
- 1 cup almond milk (or other non-dairy milk)
- 1 tablespoon maple syrup (optional)
- 1/2 teaspoon vanilla extract

- Fresh berries for topping

Instructions:

- In a bowl, combine chia seeds, almond milk, maple syrup, and vanilla extract. Stir well to avoid clumping.
- Refrigerate for at least 2 hours or overnight until it thickens.
- Serve topped with fresh berries.

These gluten-free, anti-inflammatory recipes are not only nutritious but also flavorful, making them perfect for any meal! Enjoy!

Mediterranean Diet Anti-Inflammatory Recipes

Here are some delicious Mediterranean diet recipes that are also anti-inflammatory:

1. Mediterranean Chickpea Salad:

Ingredients:

- 1 can chickpeas, rinsed and drained
- 1 cup cherry tomatoes, halved
- 1 cucumber, diced
- 1/4 red onion, finely chopped
- 1/4 cup kalamata olives, pitted and sliced
- 1/4 cup feta cheese (optional)
- 2 tablespoons olive oil
- Juice of 1 lemon
- Salt and pepper to taste
- Fresh parsley, chopped

Instructions:

- In a large bowl, combine chickpeas, tomatoes, cucumber, red onion, olives, and feta.
- In a small bowl, whisk together olive oil, lemon juice, salt, and pepper.
- Pour the dressing over the salad, toss gently, and garnish with parsley before serving.

2. Lemon Herb Grilled Chicken:

Ingredients:

- 4 chicken breasts
- 1/4 cup olive oil
- Juice of 2 lemons
- 3 cloves garlic, minced
- 1 teaspoon dried oregano
- Salt and pepper to taste

Instructions:

- In a bowl, mix olive oil, lemon juice, garlic, oregano, salt, and pepper.
- Marinate chicken breasts in the mixture for at least 30 minutes.
- Preheat the grill to medium-high heat and cook chicken for 6-7 minutes per side or until fully cooked. Serve with a side of vegetables.

3. Quinoa Tabbouleh:

Ingredients:

- 1 cup cooked quinoa
- 1 cup parsley, finely chopped
- 1/2 cup mint, finely chopped
- 1 cup cherry tomatoes, diced
- 1/4 cup red onion, finely chopped

- Juice of 1 lemon

- 2 tablespoons olive oil

- Salt and pepper to taste

Instructions:

- In a large bowl, combine cooked quinoa, parsley, mint, tomatoes, and red onion.

- In a separate bowl, whisk together lemon juice, olive oil, salt, and pepper.

- Pour dressing over the quinoa mixture and toss to combine. Chill before serving.

4. Roasted Vegetables with Balsamic Glaze:

Ingredients:

- 1 zucchini, sliced

- 1 bell pepper, diced

- 1 red onion, cut into wedges

- 1 cup cherry tomatoes

- 2 tablespoons olive oil

- Salt and pepper to taste

- Balsamic glaze for drizzling

Instructions:

- Preheat the oven to 425°F (220°C).

- Toss vegetables with olive oil, salt, and pepper on a baking sheet.

- Roast for 20-25 minutes, until tender and slightly caramelized. Drizzle with balsamic glaze before serving.

5. Greek Yogurt Parfait:

Ingredients:

- 1 cup Greek yogurt (plain, unsweetened)

- 1/2 cup mixed berries (blueberries, strawberries, raspberries)
- 1 tablespoon honey (optional)
- 1/4 cup granola (optional, choose a low-sugar variety)
- Chopped nuts for topping (optional)

Instructions:

- In a glass or bowl, layer Greek yogurt, mixed berries, and granola.
- Drizzle with honey if desired and top with chopped nuts. Enjoy as a breakfast or snack!

These Mediterranean-inspired recipes are not only flavorful but also packed with anti-inflammatory ingredients, making them perfect for a healthy diet! Enjoy!

Paleo Diet Anti-Inflammatory Recipes

Here are some tasty Paleo diet recipes that are also anti-inflammatory:

1. Paleo Lemon Garlic Chicken:

Ingredients:

- 4 chicken breasts
- 3 tablespoons olive oil
- Juice of 2 lemons
- 4 cloves garlic, minced
- 1 teaspoon dried thyme
- Salt and pepper to taste

Instructions:

- In a bowl, whisk together olive oil, lemon juice, garlic, thyme, salt, and pepper.
- Marinate chicken breasts in the mixture for at least 30 minutes.

- Preheat a skillet over medium heat and cook chicken for about 6-7 minutes per side, or until cooked through. Serve with steamed vegetables.

2. Sweet Potato and Kale Hash:

Ingredients:

- 2 large sweet potatoes, diced
- 2 cups kale, chopped
- 1 onion, diced
- 2 tablespoons olive oil
- 1 teaspoon paprika
- Salt and pepper to taste

Instructions:

- Heat olive oil in a large skillet over medium heat. Add diced sweet potatoes and onion; cook until sweet potatoes are tender, about 10-15 minutes.

- Stir in kale, paprika, salt, and pepper. Cook until kale is wilted, about 3-5 minutes. Serve warm.

3. Coconut Curry Shrimp:

Ingredients:

- 1 lb shrimp, peeled and deveined
- 1 can coconut milk
- 2 tablespoons red curry paste
- 1 cup bell peppers, sliced
- 1 tablespoon fresh ginger, minced
- 2 tablespoons olive oil
- Fresh cilantro for garnish

Instructions:

- In a large skillet, heat olive oil over medium heat. Add ginger and bell peppers; sauté for 3-4 minutes.

- Stir in coconut milk and curry paste, bringing to a simmer.

- Add shrimp and cook until pink and cooked through, about 5 minutes. Garnish with fresh cilantro before serving.

4. Zucchini Noodles with Avocado Pesto:

Ingredients:

- 2 medium zucchinis, spiralized
- 1 avocado
- 1/4 cup basil leaves
- 2 tablespoons olive oil
- Juice of 1 lemon
- Salt and pepper to taste

Instructions:

- In a food processor, combine avocado, basil, olive oil, lemon juice, salt, and pepper. Blend until smooth.

- Toss zucchini noodles with avocado pesto until well coated. Serve raw or lightly sautéed for a few minutes.

5. Baked Salmon with Asparagus:

Ingredients:

- 4 salmon fillets
- 1 bunch asparagus, trimmed
- 2 tablespoons olive oil
- Juice of 1 lemon
- Salt and pepper to taste
- Fresh dill for garnish (optional)

Instructions:

- Preheat the oven to 400°F (200°C). Line a baking sheet with parchment paper.

- Place salmon fillets and asparagus on the baking sheet. Drizzle with olive oil, lemon juice, salt, and pepper.
- Bake for 12-15 minutes, or until salmon is cooked through and asparagus is tender. Garnish with dill if desired.

These Paleo recipes are not only anti-inflammatory but also packed with flavor, making them great options for healthy meals! Enjoy!

CHAPTER SIX
Stress Management Techniques, Exercise And Physical Activity

Here are some effective stress management techniques, along with insights on exercise and physical activity:

Stress Management Techniques

Mindfulness and Meditation:

- Practice mindfulness meditation to focus on the present moment and reduce anxiety.
- Use apps or guided sessions to help you get started.

Deep Breathing Exercises:

- Engage in deep breathing techniques, such as diaphragmatic breathing, to activate the relaxation response.

- Inhale deeply through your nose, hold for a few seconds, and exhale slowly through your mouth.

Progressive Muscle Relaxation:

- Tense and relax different muscle groups in your body systematically to relieve physical tension.
- Start from your toes and work your way up to your head.

Journaling:

- Write about your thoughts and feelings to gain clarity and reduce stress.
- Consider keeping a gratitude journal to focus on positive aspects of your life.

Time Management:

- Prioritize tasks and set realistic goals to reduce feelings of overwhelm.
- Break tasks into smaller, manageable steps.

Connect with Others:

- Talk to friends, family, or support groups to share your feelings and gain perspective.
- Engage in social activities to build connections and alleviate stress.

Exercise and Physical Activity:

Regular Aerobic Exercise:

- Activities like walking, jogging, cycling, and swimming can boost mood and reduce anxiety through the release of endorphins.

- Aim for at least 150 minutes of moderate aerobic exercise per week.

Strength Training:

- Incorporate resistance exercises to improve strength and overall physical health.
- Consider activities like weightlifting, bodyweight exercises, or yoga.

Yoga and Tai Chi:

- Both practices combine movement, meditation, and breathing, promoting relaxation and stress reduction.

- Classes or online videos can guide you through poses and techniques.

Outdoor Activities:

- Spend time in nature through hiking, gardening, or simply walking in a park to enhance your mood and reduce stress.
- Nature exposure has been linked to lower stress levels and improved mental health.

Group Classes or Sports:

- Join group fitness classes, dance classes, or sports teams to combine social interaction with physical activity.
- The camaraderie can enhance motivation and enjoyment.

<u>Tips for Getting Started:</u>

- **Set Realistic Goals**: Start small and gradually increase the intensity or duration of your activities.

- **Find What You Enjoy**: Choose exercises and activities that you find fun to ensure consistency.

- **Create a Routine**: Incorporate physical activity into your daily schedule for better adherence.

By integrating stress management strategies with consistent physical activity, it is possible to enhance one's mental health and resilience to stress.

Conclusion

It is imperative to manage stress and maintain overall well-being in order to lead a healthy existence. Individuals can improve their mental and physical health by incorporating effective stress management techniques, such as mindfulness, deep breathing, and journaling, into their routines, in addition to regular exercise and physical activity.

Not only does the adoption of practices that encourage physical fitness, social connections, and relaxation alleviate tension, but it also cultivates resilience and a positive perspective on life.

A more balanced and fulfilling life can be achieved by taking proactive steps toward stress management, whether through engaging in mindful meditation or finding pleasure in outdoor activities. By prioritizing these practices, you will be able to more effectively and peacefully confront the obstacles that life presents.

THE END

www.ingramcontent.com/pod-product-compliance
Lightning Source LLC
Chambersburg PA
CBHW061100250726
48653CB00001B/494